Do You Love Your Team?

A Quiz Book
for Man City Fans

by

Matt Maguire

Publisher Information

Candescent Press
info@candescentpress.co.uk
www.candescentpress.co.uk

ISBN-13: 978-1481199148

ISBN-10: 1481199145

This book is an unofficial publication and is not authorised in any way by Manchester City Football Club.

CONTENTS

Welcome

So, you think you're a fan? Well now is the time to find out just how much you love your team. We hope we've got questions that every fan will be able to answer, alongside some that will have even the die-hard season ticket holders scratching their heads.

Get ready to find out just how much you know about Manchester City - and we hope you'll learn a few new facts to surprise your friends with!

About the Book

The book is split into nine sections, ranging from Pre-Season Training through to The Cup Final. Each section is a game of two halves!

After every ten questions you get the questions repeated along with the answers so you can quickly see how well you got on!

From the Author...

I've been a City fan all my life, and writing this book has brought back some amazing memories - and also a few frustrated ones.

I remember watching City beat Stoke 5-2 while on holiday in 1988. Just me and two Stoke fans, drifting together to the "old third division" - the rest of the bar not quite understanding why no-one was happy.

I have much happier memories of the '81 Cup Final (despite the result). My Dad took me and my sister out of school for the day, telling them that we were both ill. A plan which would have worked, had we not been featured on the local news departing Piccadilly (and waving furiously at the cameras).

Happily, we've now started to get a few more positive results on the pitch, but I still wouldn't swap any of the ups and downs - looking back, I truly love being a City fan.

I'd like to dedicate this book to my dad, who made me the fan, and the person, that I am today. He sadly passed away a couple of years ago, but I've included a couple of extra questions about his hero Tony Book as a small tribute.

CTID
Matt Maguire

1. Pre-season Training

First Half

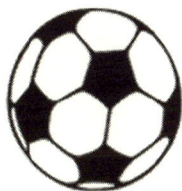

QUESTIONS

1. Born in 1953, he scored the goal that took City to Wembley in 1981. Who was he?

2. Who did City beat in the 1956 FA Cup Final?

3. From which club did City buy Georgi Kinkladze?

4. Who was the first Irish player to win City's Player of the Season award?

5. Tony Book played well over 200 games for City, but how old was he when he signed?

6. Which 2008 Olympic gold medallists went on to play for City?

7. City legend Mike Summerbee's son also played for City. What was his name?

8. Who captained City to a 1986 Youth Cup Final win over Manchester United?

9. Which outfield player saved a penalty, when Tony Coton was sent off in a 1991 league match?

10. Whose autobiography is entitled, "I'm Not Really Here"?

1. Pre-season Training

First Half

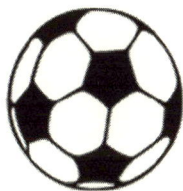

ANSWERS

1. Born in 1953, he scored the goal that took City to Wembley in 1981. Who was he?

A. **Paul Power.**

2. Who did City beat in the 1956 FA Cup Final?

A. **Birmingham City.**

3. From which club did City buy Georgi Kinkladze?

A. **Dinamo Tbilisi.**

4. Who was the first Irish player to win City's Player of the Season award?

A. **Mick McCarthy in 1984.**

5. Tony Book played well over 200 games for City, but how old was he when he signed?

A. **31.**

6. Which 2008 Olympic gold medallists went on to play for City?

A. **Pablo Zabaleta and Sergio Agüero. Argentina won the men's football gold.**

7. City legend Mike Summerbee's son also played for City. What was his name?

A. **Nicky Summerbee.**

8. Who captained City to a 1986 Youth Cup Final win over Manchester United?

A. **Steve Redmond.**

9. Which outfield player saved a penalty, when Tony Coton was sent off in a 1991 league match?

A. **Niall Quinn. At the time clubs rarely named a sub goalkeeper.**

10. Whose autobiography is entitled, "I'm Not Really Here"?

A. **Paul Lake.**

1. Pre-season Training

Second Half

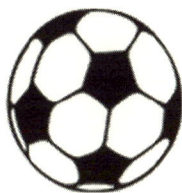

QUESTIONS

11. In 2004 City famously came back from 3-0 down (with ten men, as Joey Barton has been sent off) to beat Spurs 4-3. Who scored the winner?

12. At which London club's former ground did City play in the 1904 FA Cup Final?

13. What nationality was early City legend Billy Meredith?

14. Which City Player of the Season winner was known as Superman?

15. Who did City beat on the final day of the season, to win the 1967/8 League Championship?

16. Three of England's 1982 World Cup Squad went on to manage City. Who were they?

17. What was the name of City's big budget documentary charting the highs and lows of the 2009/10 season?

18. Which ex-city player died in the Munich air disaster?

19. "Feed the Goat and He Will Score" - who was The Goat?

20. What ground did City play at before Maine Road?

1. Pre-season Training

Second Half

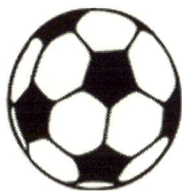

ANSWERS

11. In 2004 City famously came back from 3-0 down (with ten men, as Joey Barton has been sent off) to beat Spurs 4-3. Who scored the winner?

A. **John Macken.**

12. At which London club's former ground did City play in the 1904 FA Cup Final?

A. **Crystal Palace.**

13. What nationality was early City legend Billy Meredith?

A. **Welsh.**

14. Which City Player of the Season winner was known as Superman?

A. **Steven Ireland.**

15. Who did City beat on the final day of the season, to win the 1967/8 League Championship?

A. **Newcastle United.**

16. Three of England's 1982 World Cup Squad went on to manage City. Who were they?

A. **Kevin Keegan, Steve Coppell, and Phil Neal (who was caretaker manager after Coppell resigned).**

17. What was the name of City's big budget documentary charting the highs and lows of the 2009/10 season?

A. **Blue Moon Rising.**

18. Which ex-city player died in the Munich air disaster?

A. **Frank Swift - he was working as a journalist and reporting on the United match.**

19. "Feed the Goat and He Will Score" - who was The Goat?

A. **Shaun Goater.**

20. What ground did City play at before Maine Road?

A. **Hyde Road.**

2. Friendly Matches

First Half

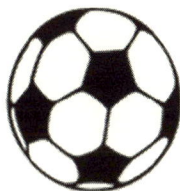

1. Born in August 1900, he played over 300 times for City, before going on to play for both Liverpool and Everton. Who was he?

2. Who said this about City, "Sometimes we're good and sometimes we're bad but when we're good, at least we're much better than we used to be and when we are bad we're just as bad as we always used to be, so that's got to be good hasn't it?"

3. Who was said to have signed 'almost by accident', after stopping off at City for a 'bite to eat', following an unsuccessful trial at Sunderland?

4. By what name is famous City fan Edward McGinnis better know?

5. Ian and David Brightwell played for City in the 90s - who were their Olympic medal winning parents?

6. City and Chelsea were involved in a nine-goal Wembley Final in 1986. What was the competition?

7. City beat Huddersfield 10-1 in 1987, but how many times did the teams play that season?

8. As of 2011, only three players have won consecutive City Player of the Season awards. Who were they?

9. City retired which shirt number following the tragic death of Marc-Vivien Foé?

10. Which City player was banned in 1905 for allegedly trying to bribe an opponent?

2. Friendly Matches

First Half

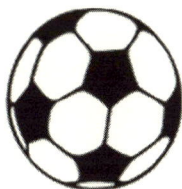

ANSWERS

1. Born in August 1900, he played over 300 times for City, before going on to play for both Liverpool and Everton. Who was he?

A. **Tommy Johnson.**

2. Who said this about City, "Sometimes we're good and sometimes we're bad but when we're good, at least we're much better than we used to be and when we are bad we're just as bad as we always used to be, so that's got to be good hasn't it?"

A. **Mark Radcliffe, BBC Radio DJ.**

3. Who was said to have signed 'almost by accident', after stopping off at City for a 'bite to eat', following an unsuccessful trial at Sunderland?

A. **Ali Benarbia.**

4. By what name is famous City fan Edward McGinnis better know?

A. **Eddie Large (of comedy duo Little and Large).**

5. Ian and David Brightwell played for City in the 90s - who were their Olympic medal winning parents?

A. **Robbie Brightwell and Ann Packer.**

6. City and Chelsea were involved in a nine-goal Wembley Final in 1986. What was the competition?

A. **The Full Members Cup. Sadly City lost, despite three goals in the last five minutes.**

7. City beat Huddersfield 10-1 in 1987, but how many times did the teams play that season?

A. **Five. City lost 1-0 in the return league fixture, but triumphed after two replays in the third round of the FA Cup.**

8. As of 2011, only three players have won consecutive City Player of the Season awards. Who were they?

A. **Mike Summerbee (1972 and 1973), Georgi Kinkladze (1996 and 1997), and Richard Dunne (2005 to 2008)**

9. City retired which shirt number following the tragic death of Marc-Vivien Foé?

A. **23. Foé died will playing for Cameroon, and had worn the number 23 shirt the previous season while on loan at City.**

10. Which City player was banned in 1905 for allegedly trying to bribe an opponent?

A. **Billy Meredith.**

2. Friendly Matches

Second Half

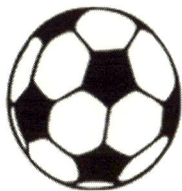

11. Who scored the opening goal in the 1976 League Cup Final?

12. Which player scored two goals for England in the 1934 'Battle of Highbury' against World Champions Italy?

13. For which Argentinian club did Georgi Kinkladze play briefly on loan?

14. The 1968/9 Football Writers' Association Player of the Year award was shared by Dave Mackay and which City player?

15. Who did City beat in the 1934 FA Cup Final, and what was the score?

16. Which relatively unknown band recorded the 'noisy' version of Blue Moon, which was often played before City matches?

17. Who played fictional footballer Sid Harmor, in the 1981 Sylvester Stallone film Escape to Victory?

18. At which English team did Uwe Rösler take over as manager in 2011?

19. Who scored for England within twenty minutes of making his debut on 18th August 2004?

20. Which ex-city goalkeeper returned to the club in 1990 to run the community programme?

2. Friendly Matches

Second Half

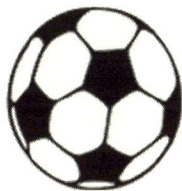

ANSWERS

11. Who scored the opening goal in the 1976 League Cup Final?

A. **Peter Barnes.**

12. Which player scored two goals for England in the 1934 'Battle of Highbury' against World Champions Italy?

A. **Eric Brook - England won 3-2.**

13. For which Argentinian club did Georgi Kinkladze play briefly on loan?

A. **Boca Juniors.**

14. The 1968/9 Football Writers' Association Player of the Year award was shared by Dave Mackay and which City player?

A. **Tony Book.**

15. Who did City beat in the 1934 FA Cup Final, and what was the score?

A. **Portsmouth. The score was 2-1.**

16. Which relatively unknown band recorded the 'noisy' version of Blue Moon, which was often played before City matches?

A. **Supra.**

17. Who played fictional footballer Sid Harmor, in the 1981 Sylvester Stallone film Escape to Victory?

A. **Mike Summerbee. Kazimierz Deyna also had a part in the film.**

18. At which English team did Uwe Rösler take over as manager in 2011?

A. **Brentford.**

19. Who scored for England within twenty minutes of making his debut on 18th August 2004?

A. **Shaun Wright-Phillips.**

20. Which ex-city goalkeeper returned to the club in 1990 to run the community programme?

A. **Alex Williams.**

3. The Season Kicks Off

First Half

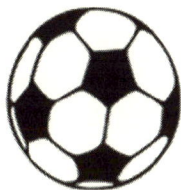

1. David Pleat famously danced across the pitch when Luton relegated City in 1983. Which future city manager played for Luton that day?

2. In what year did Man City move to Maine Road?

3. Who managed City to their first League Championship win in 1937?

4. Every player in City's European Cup Winner's Cup winning team was English . True or False?

5. Who did City pay Queens Park Rangers £200,000 for in 1972?

6. Which three players scored City's goals in their 1956 FA Cup Final win?

7. Which Liverpudlian had two spells with City, before heading off to the sun with the Miami Fusion.

8. Who is the Japanese cartoon character that gave Sergio Agüero his nickname?

9. How many times have City won the Charity Shield?

10. What was the name of the restaurant that Colin Bell co-owned with another footballer Colin Waldron?

3. The Season Kicks Off

First Half

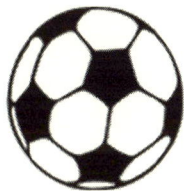

ANSWERS

1. David Pleat famously danced across the pitch when Luton relegated City in 1983. Which future city manager played for Luton that day?

A. **Brian Horton.**

2. In what year did Man City move to Maine Road?

A. **1923.**

3. Who managed City to their first League Championship win in 1937?

A. **Wilf Wild.**

4. Every player in City's European Cup Winner's Cup winning team was English . True or False?

A. **True. Even the sub and manager were English.**

5. Who did City pay Queens Park Rangers £200,000 for in 1972?

A. **Rodney Marsh.**

6. Which three players scored City's goals in their 1956 FA Cup Final win?

A. **Joe Hayes, Jack Dyson and Bobby Johnstone.**

7. Which Liverpudlian had two spells with City, before heading off to the sun with the Miami Fusion.

A. **Ian Bishop.**

8. Who is the Japanese cartoon character that gave Sergio Agüero his nickname?

A. **Kum Kum**

9. How many times have City won the Charity Shield?

A. **Three. In 1937, 1968 and 1972.**

10. What was the name of the restaurant that Colin Bell co-owned with another footballer Colin Waldron?

A. **The Bell Waldron.**

3. The Season Kicks Off

Second Half

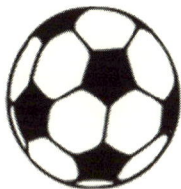

11. What nationality was City legend Bert Trautmann?

12. Which team did did Sven-Göran Eriksson manage after leaving City?

13. Who did Alan Ball say would be the first British £10 million pound player?

14. Who scored both City's goals in the 1934 FA Cup Final win?

15. City broke the British transfer record in 1979 to buy Steve Daley from which club?

16. The highest attendance at any English football match was at Maine Road in 1934. 84,569 people attended, and saw City play which team?

17. What nationality is Edin Džeko?

18. Which City player won the PFA Young Player Of The Year award in 1976?

19. He was England's first ever million pound footballer, and later went on to play for City. Who was he?

20. Whose 'day' is celebrated on the 21st June each year?

3. The Season Kicks Off

Second Half

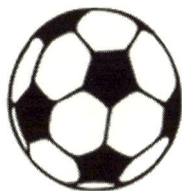

ANSWERS

11. What nationality was City legend Bert Trautmann?

A. **German.**

12. Which team did did Sven-Göran Eriksson manage after leaving City?

A. **The Mexico national team.**

13. Who did Alan Ball say would be the first British £10 million pound player?

A. **Martin 'Buster' Phillips. He wasn't.**

14. Who scored both City's goals in the 1934 FA Cup Final win?

A. **Fred Tilson.**

15. City broke the British transfer record in 1979 to buy Steve Daley from which club?

A. **Wolverhampton Wanderers.**

16. The highest attendance at any English football match was at Maine Road in 1934. 84,569 people attended, and saw City play which team?

A. **Stoke, in the FA Cup sixth round.**

17. What nationality is Edin Džeko?

A. **Bosnian.**

18. Which City player won the PFA Young Player Of The Year award in 1976?

A. **Peter Barnes.**

19. He was England's first ever million pound footballer, and later went on to play for City. Who was he?

A. **Trevor Francis. He was bought for £1m by Notts Forest - two years later he joined City.**

20. Whose 'day' is celebrated on the 21st June each year?

A. **The 21st is known as 'Shaun Goater Day' in Bermuda.**

4. The Early Leaders

First Half

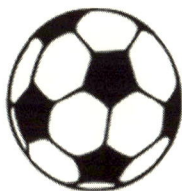

1. Who did City beat in the very first public match at the City of Manchester (now Etihad) Stadium?

2. Carlos Tévez made his debut for which club in 2001?

3. Which City manager was known as the 'Footballing Grocer'?

4. Which three players scored hat-tricks in City's famous 10-1 win against Huddersfield?

5. What are the names of Manchester City's lunar mascots?

6. Who did City beat to win their first FA Cup?

7. With what fruit did City start the 1987 football inflatables craze?

8. Whose wife apparently said, "You love Malcolm Allison more than you love me"?

9. Which player famously danced in his Disco Pants?

10. Who was Kinky?

4. The Early Leaders

First Half

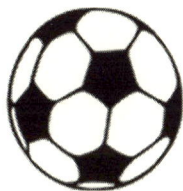

ANSWERS

1. Who did City beat in the very first public match at the City of Manchester (now Etihad) Stadium?

A. **Barcelona - 2-1.**

2. Carlos Tévez made his debut for which club in 2001?

A. **Boca Juniors.**

3. Which City manager was known as the 'Footballing Grocer'?

A. **Joe Mercer. He ran a grocery store during his playing career.**

4. Which three players scored hat-tricks in City's famous 10-1 win against Huddersfield?

A. **Paul Stewart, Tony Adcock and David White.**

5. What are the names of Manchester City's lunar mascots?

A. **Moonchester and Moonbeam.**

6. Who did City beat to win their first FA Cup?

A. **Bolton Wanderers.**

7. With what fruit did City start the 1987 football inflatables craze?

A. **The inflatable banana!**

8. Whose wife apparently said, "You love Malcolm Allison more than you love me"?

A. **Mike Summerbee's.**

9. Which player famously danced in his Disco Pants?

A. **Niall Quinn.**

10. Who was Kinky?

A. **Georgi Kinkladze.**

4. The Early Leaders

Second Half

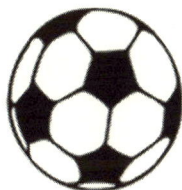

11. Who managed City to consecutive fifth place finishes in the early 1990s?

12. Who did City play in their first league game at Maine Road?

13. Who was voted 1999 UNPF Player of the Year in the French first division?

14. For which team did City manager Joe Mercer play the most games?

15. Who scored the last competitive goal at Maine Road, and for which team?

16. Who scored the first competitive goal at City's current stadium?

17. Who suggested in 2003 that Kevin Keegan had behaved "like a big baby"?

18. Who captained City in their 1976 League Cup Final win?

19. Between 2008 and 2010, City signed three Hamburg first team players. Who were they?

20. In what year did City play their last match at Maine Road?

4. The Early Leaders

Second Half

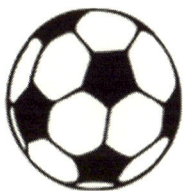

ANSWERS

11. Who managed City to consecutive fifth place finishes in the early 1990s?

A. **Peter Reid.**

12. Who did City play in their first league game at Maine Road?

A. **Sheffield United.**

13. Who was voted 1999 UNPF Player of the Year in the French first division?

A. **Ali Benarbia.**

14. For which team did City manager Joe Mercer play the most games?

A. **Arsenal.**

15. Who scored the last competitive goal at Maine Road, and for which team?

A. **Michael Svensson for Southampton in a 1-0 defeat.**

16. Who scored the first competitive goal at City's current stadium?

A. **Trevor Sinclair in a UEFA Cup qualifying match against TNS.**

17. Who suggested in 2003 that Kevin Keegan had behaved "like a big baby"?

A. **Eyal Berkovic.**

18. Who captained City in their 1976 League Cup Final win?

A. **Mike Doyle.**

19. Between 2008 and 2010, City signed three Hamburg first team players. Who were they?

A. **Vincent Kompany, Nigel de Jong and Jérôme Boateng.**

20. In what year did City play their last match at Maine Road?

A. **2003.**

5. The Busy Xmas Period

First Half

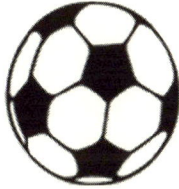

QUESTIONS

1. In 1967 City won a match in atrocious weather, which became known as the 'Ballet On Ice'. Who did they beat?

2. Which City player made his debut in 1962, aged just 15?

3. Kiki Musampa, played for City from 2004-06, but an urban myth arose that he had a brother. What was the fictional brother called?

4. In the 1950s two City players won the Football Writers' Association Player of the Year award. Who were they?

5. City won the 1970 Cup Winner's Cup Final in which country?

6. John Bond signed two moustachioed players who took part in the 1981 FA Cup Final. Who were they?

7. Who captained City in September 2007 against Aston Villa, aged just 19?

8. From which team did City buy Colin Bell?

9. City reached the FA Cup Final twice in the fifties, who was their manager for both matches?

10. Who did City beat in the 1970 League Cup Final?

5. The Busy Xmas Period

First Half

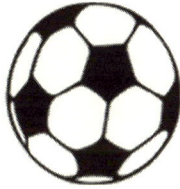

ANSWERS

1. In 1967 City won a match in atrocious weather, which became known as the 'Ballet On Ice'. Who did they beat?

A. **Tottenham Hotspur.**

2. Which City player made his debut in 1962, aged just 15?

A. **Glyn Pardoe.**

3. Kiki Musampa, played for City from 2004-06, but an urban myth arose that he had a brother. What was the fictional brother called?

A. **Kris Musampa (as in Christmas Hamper).**

4. In the 1950s two City players won the Football Writers' Association Player of the Year award. Who were they?

A. **Don Revie (in 1955) and Bert Trautmann (in 1956).**

5. City won the 1970 Cup Winner's Cup Final in which country?

A. **Austria - the game was played in Vienna.**

6. John Bond signed two moustachioed players who took part in the 1981 FA Cup Final. Who were they?

A. **Gerry Gow and Tommy Hutchison.**

7. Who captained City in September 2007 against Aston Villa, aged just 19?

A. **Micah Richards.**

8. From which team did City buy Colin Bell?

A. **Bury.**

9. City reached the FA Cup Final twice in the fifties, who was their manager for both matches?

A. **Les McDowell.**

10. Who did City beat in the 1970 League Cup Final?

A. **West Bromwich Albion.**

5. The Busy Xmas Period

Second Half

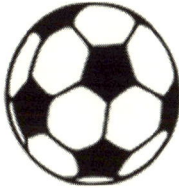

QUESTIONS

11. Who scored City's opening goal in the 1989 5-1 Manchester derby win?

12. Which City player was offered a contract by an Australian Rules team before he decided on a career in football?

13. What was the original proposed capacity of Maine Road - 90, 100, or 120 thousand?

14. At which club did Vincent Kompany start his career?

15. From which club was Joe Hart signed?

16. Francis Lee scored so many penalties, that he earned what nickname?

17. "He trains at 25 per cent, if it was 50 per cent he could be one of the world's best players" - who was talking, and which player was he referring to?

18. What was the Kippax stand at Maine Road, formerly known as?

19. When did City first play in the Charity Shield at Wembley? 1934, 1968, or 2011?

20. What is the name of the hat that title winning City coach Malcolm Allison famously wore?

5. The Busy Xmas Period

Second Half

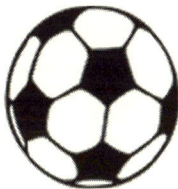

ANSWERS

11. Who scored City's opening goal in the 1989 5-1 Manchester derby win?

A. **David Oldfield.**

12. Which City player was offered a contract by an Australian Rules team before he decided on a career in football?

A. **Niall Quinn.**

13. What was the original proposed capacity of Maine Road - 90, 100, or 120 thousand?

A. **120 thousand. Unfortunately these plans were scaled back.**

14. At which club did Vincent Kompany start his career?

A. **Anderlecht.**

15. From which club was Joe Hart signed?

A. **Shrewsbury Town.**

16. Francis Lee scored so many penalties, that he earned what nickname?

A. **Lee One Pen.**

17. "He trains at 25 per cent, if it was 50 per cent he could be one of the world's best players" - who was talking, and which player was he referring to?

A. **Jose Mourinho talking about Mario Balotelli, when they were both at Inter.**

18. What was the Kippax stand at Maine Road, formerly known as?

A. **The Popular Side.**

19. When did City first play in the Charity Shield at Wembley? 1934, 1968, or 2011?

A. **2011. This was their eighth Charity Shield, but the first they played at Wembley.**

20. What is the name of the hat that title winning City coach Malcolm Allison famously wore?

A. **The Fedora.**

6. Mid-season Madness

First Half

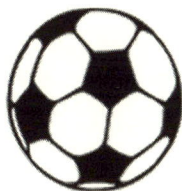

QUESTIONS

1. Which woman is considered to be Man City's founder?

2. As of 2011, how many City players had won the PFA Player of the Year award?

3. The venue was the City of Manchester Stadium, the date, 2005, the opponents Finland. Carney scores for England. What was the tournament?

4. Which national team did Uwe Rösler play for?

5. Who said this about City hero Georgi Kinkladze: "I couldn't help deducing that contrary to popular opinion, he would be my weak link not my strong one."?

6. Against which team did Adam Johnson score his first international goal?

7. Which two City players represented England at the 1970 World Cup Finals?

8. Following their league championship, City won the '68 Charity Shield 6-1. Who did they beat?

9. From which team did City buy David Silva?

10. In what year did City win their first League Championship?

6. Mid-season Madness

First Half

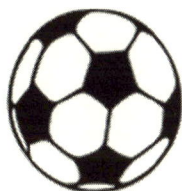

ANSWERS

1. Which woman is considered to be Man City's founder?

A. **Anne Connell.**

2. As of 2011, how many City players had won the PFA Player of the Year award?

A. **None.**

3. The venue was the City of Manchester Stadium, the date, 2005, the opponents Finland. Carney scores for England. What was the tournament?

A. **UEFA Women's Euro 2005.**

4. Which national team did Uwe Rösler play for?

A. **East Germany - he played just before the East and West German teams were unified.**

5. Who said this about City hero Georgi Kinkladze: "I couldn't help deducing that contrary to popular opinion, he would be my weak link not my strong one."?

A. **Joe Royle.**

6. Against which team did Adam Johnson score his first international goal?

A. **Bulgaria. In a Euro 2012 qualifier on 3rd September 2010.**

7. Which two City players represented England at the 1970 World Cup Finals?

A. **Colin Bell and Francis Lee.**

8. Following their league championship, City won the '68 Charity Shield 6-1. Who did they beat?

A. **West Bromwich Albion.**

9. From which team did City buy David Silva?

A. **Valencia.**

10. In what year did City win their first League Championship?

A. **1937.**

6. Mid-season Madness

Second Half

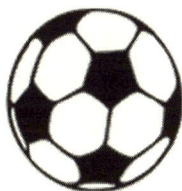

QUESTIONS

11. What nationality was 70s star, Kazimierz Deyna?

12. What is Elano's middle name?

13. Which City team did Tony Book play more games for, Bath or Manchester?

14. Which player captained City in the 1999 2nd Division play-off final?

15. Who is City's all time top goalscorer?

16. What number was David Silva given when he joined City?

17. Who scored City's winning goal in the 1969 FA Cup Final?

18. Whose name is tattooed on Sergio Agüero's right arm?

19. What nationality are Yaya and Kolo Touré?

20. Which two players scored the goals for City, in the 1970 Cup Winner's Cup Final?

6. Mid-season Madness

Second Half

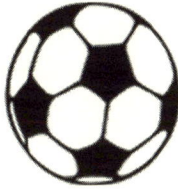

ANSWERS

11. What nationality was 70s star, Kazimierz Deyna?

A. **Polish.**

12. What is Elano's middle name?

A. **He hasn't got one. He explained in a 2007 interview with the Guardian that he has no idea why people think his middle name is Ralph.**

13. Which City team did Tony Book play more games for, Bath or Manchester?

A. **Bath City - he played over 100 more games for them.**

14. Which player captained City in the 1999 2nd Division play-off final?

A. **Andy Morrison.**

15. Who is City's all time top goalscorer?

A. **Eric Brook.**

16. What number was David Silva given when he joined City?

A. **21.**

17. Who scored City's winning goal in the 1969 FA Cup Final?

A. **Neil Young.**

18. Whose name is tattooed on Sergio Agüero's right arm?

A. **His own name (and nickname) - Kun Agüero.**

19. What nationality are Yaya and Kolo Touré?

A. **Ivorian (from Côte d'Ivoire).**

20. Which two players scored the goals for City, in the 1970 Cup Winner's Cup Final?

A. **Neil Young and Francis Lee.**

7. The Business End

First Half

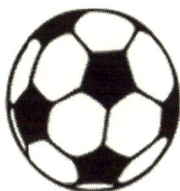

QUESTIONS

1. Who did Tony Book replace as City manager in 1974?

2. In 1937/8 City were top scorers in the First Division. What was unusual about that fact?

3. In 1999 who mistakenly said "Looks like Scunny next year"?

4. As of 2011, only one Ballon d'Or winner had ever played for City. Who was he?

5. From which club did City sign Francis Lee?

6. Who scored City's winner in the 1976 League Cup Final?

7. Which goalkeeper has made most appearances for City?

8. What were City legend Colin Bell's two main nicknames?

9. Who did Man City beat in the 2008 Youth Cup Final?

10. City won the 1970 League Cup Final 2-1. Who scored City's goals?

7. The Business End

First Half

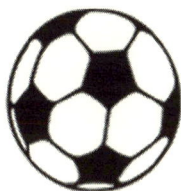

ANSWERS

1. Who did Tony Book replace as City manager in 1974?

A. **Ron Saunders.**

2. In 1937/8 City were top scorers in the First Division. What was unusual about that fact?

A. **City were relegated despite scoring more goals than every other team that year.**

3. In 1999 who mistakenly said "Looks like Scunny next year"?

A. **Joe Royle, when City were 2-0 down in the 2nd Division play-off final.**

4. As of 2011, only one Ballon d'Or winner had ever played for City. Who was he?

A. **George Weah. He won the prize in 1995 and played for City in 2000.**

5. From which club did City sign Francis Lee?

A. **Bolton Wanderers.**

6. Who scored City's winner in the 1976 League Cup Final?

A. **Dennis Tueart, with a stunning overhead kick.**

7. Which goalkeeper has made most appearances for City?

A. **Joe Corrigan.**

8. What were City legend Colin Bell's two main nicknames?

A. **Colin the King (or King of the Kippax), and Nijinsky (after the racehorse).**

9. Who did Man City beat in the 2008 Youth Cup Final?

A. **Chelsea. City won 4-2 on aggregate.**

10. City won the 1970 League Cup Final 2-1. Who scored City's goals?

A. **Mike Doyle and Glyn Pardoe.**

7. The Business End

Second Half

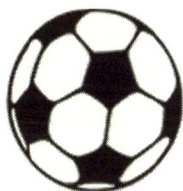

QUESTIONS

11. There are three teams that Sven-Göran Eriksson and Roberto Mancini have both managed. Name them.

12. Why was an area at Maine Road known as the Gene Kelly stand?

13. As of 2011, how many times had City been English League Champions?

14. Whose goal for City relegated Manchester United in the 1973/74 season.

15. From which club did City sign Shaun Goater?

16. City had a fifty-fifty chance of facing Roma in the 1970 Cup Winner's Cup Final. Why?

17. Joe Hart won the Premier League Golden Glove in 2011. How many clean sheets did he keep to win it?

18. In the 1980s three future City managers won the PFA Player of the Year award. Who were they?

19. Which former City captain was sent off for 'sticking his tongue out' at Stan Collymore?

20. Which player scored for City on his debut against Chelsea in 2008?

7. The Business End

Second Half

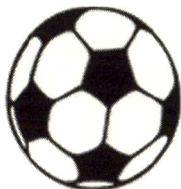

ANSWERS

11. There are three teams that Sven-Göran Eriksson and Roberto Mancini have both managed. Name them.

A. **Lazio, Fiorentina, and, of course, Manchester City.**

12. Why was an area at Maine Road known as the Gene Kelly stand?

A. **The section in the corner of the ground had no roof, and Gene Kelly famously sang "Singing in the Rain".**

13. As of 2011, how many times had City been English League Champions?

A. **Twice.**

14. Whose goal for City relegated Manchester United in the 1973/74 season.

A. **Denis Law. The goal meant it was impossible for United to stay up, no matter what results were elsewhere.**

15. From which club did City sign Shaun Goater?

A. **Bristol City.**

16. City had a fifty-fifty chance of facing Roma in the 1970 Cup Winner's Cup Final. Why?

A. **Because the Semi-final between Górnik Zabrze and Roma ended in a draw, and was decided by a coin toss. Each team had exactly a 50% chance of winning the coin toss.**

17. Joe Hart won the Premier League Golden Glove in 2011. How many clean sheets did he keep to win it?

A. **18.**

18. In the 1980s three future City managers won the PFA Player of the Year award. Who were they?

A. **Kevin Keegan (1982), Peter Reid ('85), and Mark Hughes ('89).**

19. Which former City captain was sent off for 'sticking his tongue out' at Stan Collymore?

A. **Andy Morrison.**

20. Which player scored for City on his debut against Chelsea in 2008?

A. **Robinho.**

8. Last Day Drama

First Half

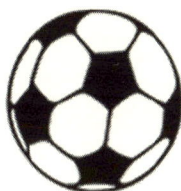

QUESTIONS

1. Roberto Mancini has only played for one club that hasn't been managed by Sven-Göran Eriksson. Which club?

2. Who captained City to their first major trophy, the 1904 FA Cup?

3. Which City manager called the club a "football factory"?

4. City won their first League Championship in 1937. Who came second?

5. Who scored City's winning goal in the 2011 FA Cup Final?

6. Which City fan is said to have coined the phrase 'The Beautiful Game'?

7. Who did City beat in the 1969 FA Cup Final?

8. How many league goals did Uwe Rösler score in his first full season at City? 12, 15, or 18?

9. In 2001, which Australian player scored one of City's finest ever individual goals, only to see it incorrectly ruled out for offside?

10. Which player scored both goals in the 1981 FA Cup final 1-1 draw?

8. Last Day Drama

First Half

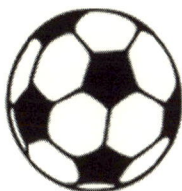

ANSWERS

1. Roberto Mancini has only played for one club that hasn't been managed by Sven-Göran Eriksson. Which club?

A. **Bologna. Sven managed Mancini's three other clubs, Sampdoria, Lazio and Leicester City.**

2. Who captained City to their first major trophy, the 1904 FA Cup?

A. **Billy Meredith.**

3. Which City manager called the club a "football factory"?

A. **Mark Hughes.**

4. City won their first League Championship in 1937. Who came second?

A. **Charlton Athletic.**

5. Who scored City's winning goal in the 2011 FA Cup Final?

A. **Yaya Touré.**

6. Which City fan is said to have coined the phrase 'The Beautiful Game'?

A. **Stuart Hall. The BBC presenter first used the term to describe the way Peter Doherty played for City.**

7. Who did City beat in the 1969 FA Cup Final?

A. **Leicester City.**

8. How many league goals did Uwe Rösler score in his first full season at City? 12, 15, or 18?

A. **15. A feat he repeated two years later in the 96/97 season.**

9. In 2001, which Australian player scored one of City's finest ever individual goals, only to see it incorrectly ruled out for offside?

A. **Danny Tiatto.**

10. Which player scored both goals in the 1981 FA Cup final 1-1 draw?

A. **Tommy Hutchison. He scored for City, then scored a freak late own goal for Spurs.**

8. Last Day Drama

Second Half

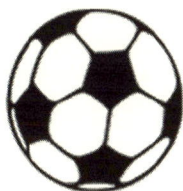

QUESTIONS

11. Was City legend Mike Doyle ever capped for England?

12. Who managed City to their first FA Cup Final win in 1904?

13. Which two players scored late goals to rescue City in the 1999 2nd Division play-off Final?

14. Glyn Pardoe played over 300 games for City, but which other clubs did he play for?

15. As of August 2011, which City manager has the highest percentage of wins?

16. Who did City beat in the 1970 European Cup Winners Cup final?

17. What Church gave City their original name?

18. Until Sven-Göran Eriksson, City had only been managed by men from which two countries?

19. Before City, Bert Trautmann played football for which town, better known for their rugby league team?

20. In which year did City win their first League Cup?

8. Last Day Drama

Second Half

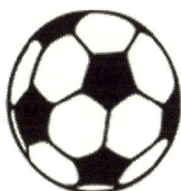

ANSWERS

11. Was City legend Mike Doyle ever capped for England?

A. **Yes. He played a handful of games in the mid-70s.**

12. Who managed City to their first FA Cup Final win in 1904?

A. **Tom Maley.**

13. Which two players scored late goals to rescue City in the 1999 2nd Division play-off Final?

A. **Kevin Horlock and Paul Dickov.**

14. Glyn Pardoe played over 300 games for City, but which other clubs did he play for?

A. **None. Glyn only played for Manchester City.**

15. As of August 2011, which City manager has the highest percentage of wins?

A. **Sam Cowan, who won two-thirds of all his games as manager.**

16. Who did City beat in the 1970 European Cup Winners Cup final?

A. **Górnik Zabrze.**

17. What Church gave City their original name?

A. **St Marks (West Gorton).**

18. Until Sven-Göran Eriksson, City had only been managed by men from which two countries?

A. **England and Scotland.**

19. Before City, Bert Trautmann played football for which town, better known for their rugby league team?

A. **St Helens.**

20. In which year did City win their first League Cup?

A. **1970.**

9. The Cup Final

First Half

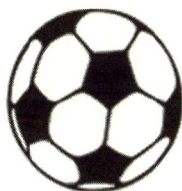

QUESTIONS

1. City were bought in 2008 by a Sheikh from which of the United Arab Emirates?

2. Between August and December 1996, five men managed or caretaker-managed City. Name them all.

3. City won the 2011 FA Cup Final, but who did they play in the third round?

4. Joe Mercer once said, "We won the League, the FA Cup, the Cup Winners' Cup and the League Cup - the only thing we didn't win was ...." What didn't City win?

5. Which Brazilian scored for City in the 2007 Manchester derby?

6. What colour shirts did City wear in the 1976 League Cup Final?

7. He played over 200 times for City, yet his statue is outside Old Trafford. Who is he?

8. City reached the League Cup Final three times, losing just once. In which year, and to which team, did they lose?

9. Who did City play in their first ever European Cup match?

10. Who managed City to their 1976 League Cup win?

9. The Cup Final

First Half

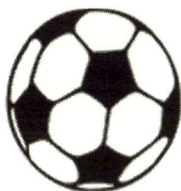

ANSWERS

1. City were bought in 2008 by a Sheikh from which of the United Arab Emirates?

A. **Abu Dhabi.**

2. Between August and December 1996, five men managed or caretaker-managed City. Name them all.

A. **Alan Ball, Asa Hartford, Steve Coppell, Phil Neal and Frank Clarke.**

3. City won the 2011 FA Cup Final, but who did they play in the third round?

A. **Leicester City.**

4. Joe Mercer once said, "We won the League, the FA Cup, the Cup Winners' Cup and the League Cup - the only thing we didn't win was ...." What didn't City win?

A. **The Grand National horse race.**

5. Which Brazilian scored for City in the 2007 Manchester derby?

A. **Geovanni.**

6. What colour shirts did City wear in the 1976 League Cup Final?

A. **Blue, they wore red and black in the 1970 Final.**

7. He played over 200 times for City, yet his statue is outside Old Trafford. Who is he?

A. **Matt Busby.**

8. City reached the League Cup Final three times, losing just once. In which year, and to which team, did they lose?

A. **1974, to Wolverhampton Wanderers.**

9. Who did City play in their first ever European Cup match?

A. **Fenerbahce.**

10. Who managed City to their 1976 League Cup win?

A. **Tony Book.**

9. The Cup Final

Second Half

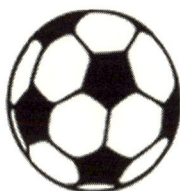

QUESTIONS

11. What do ex-City players Paul Futcher and Jeff Whitley have in common?

12. Manchester City were formed in the 1890s. What were they known as just before that date?

13. Who scored a wonder goal for City in the 1981 FA Cup Final replay?

14. For what sporting event was the Etihad Stadium originally built?

15. When Uwe Rösler left City, he joined which German club?

16. Which two Man City players were in England's 1982 World Cup squad?

17. In the year City won their first top division title, where did Manchester United finish?

18. Who are the only two players to have scored more than 150 league goals for City?

19. Which club beat City in the 1933 FA Cup Final?

20. Dennis Tueart had two spells as a player at City. Which US team did he play for in between?

9. The Cup Final

Second Half

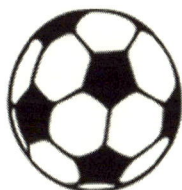

ANSWERS

11. What do ex-City players Paul Futcher and Jeff Whitley have in common?

A. **They both had brothers who played for City (Ron and Jim respectively).**

12. Manchester City were formed in the 1890s. What were they known as just before that date?

A. **Ardwick AFC.**

13. Who scored a wonder goal for City in the 1981 FA Cup Final replay?

A. **Steve MacKenzie.**

14. For what sporting event was the Etihad Stadium originally built?

A. **The 2002 Commonwealth Games.**

15. When Uwe Rösler left City, he joined which German club?

A. **FC Kaiserslautern.**

16. Which two Man City players were in England's 1982 World Cup squad?

A. **Trevor Francis and Joe Corrigan.**

17. In the year City won their first top division title, where did Manchester United finish?

A. **They were relegated after finishing in 21st place.**

18. Who are the only two players to have scored more than 150 league goals for City?

A. **Eric Brook and Tommy Johnson.**

19. Which club beat City in the 1933 FA Cup Final?

A. **Everton.**

20. Dennis Tueart had two spells as a player at City. Which US team did he play for in between?

A. **New York Cosmos.**

Congratulations!

If you've reached this far, and learnt a few new facts, then you officially love City.

Thanks for buying the book. We really hope you enjoyed it, and if you have any comments, questions, or suggestions please contact us at info@candescentpress.co.uk

We believe all the answers are correct as of September 2011, but if you fancy challenging our knowledge let us know on the above email.

Matt Maguire
The Candescent Press

Printed in Great Britain
by Amazon.co.uk, Ltd.,
Marston Gate.